Yoga for Chronic Pain

*7 steps to aid recovery
from fibromyalgia with yoga*

Kayla Kurin

Yoga for Chronic Pain: 7 Steps to Aid Recovery From Fibromyalgia with Yoga by Kayla Kurin.

www.arogayoga.com

© 2018 Kayla Kurin

info@arogayoga.com

Cover photography: CC0 public domain
Book photography: Sarah Bouchard

Other Books By Kayla Kurin

Yoga for Chronic Fatigue

Yoga for Insomnia

Where Can I Find Wifi? Work Anywhere,
Travel Forever: Tales of a Digital Nomad

Contents

Dear reader,

How are you feeling right now? On a scale of 1-10?

Can I guess that you are somewhere on the pain side of things? Can I also imagine that your pain isn't going away? Whether you take medication, go to what feels like hundreds of doctors appointments, go for walks in nature, or rest – the next day, you're still in pain. How many times has someone promised you they could fix it if you have a few thousand dollars to fork over, but you've still come out feeling the same?

I wish I could reach out of the pages of this book and give you a great big hug because I know how it feels to be in terrible pain. For years, I woke up in pain and was exhausted all day. Even worse, no doctor could tell me how to fix it. I tried so many different things: doctors, naturopaths, sleeping pills and supplements that tasted like dirt. Sometimes, the medication would work for a time, but mostly, it was just covering up the problem. I went on like this for years, feeling like I was only living half a life.

Despite some people thinking I was depressed or just lazy, I wanted to be doing the things my friends were doing. I wanted to be playing sports, attending classes, and travelling. But I couldn't do any of it, no matter what I tried.

After I had been living with illness for almost 7 years, someone recommended I try yoga. I said no. I didn't think it would work for me. I felt that my illness was serious, and yoga was better suited to people who were a bit stressed out or looking for a new way to exercise. Then, another person recommended I try meditation. I also said no. If a doctor couldn't help me, I had no idea how a few breathing exercises would do anything. Instead, I continued bouncing between doctors and trying different medications. Finally, after my seven year anniversary with the illness, I picked up a yoga DVD. It couldn't hurt, could it?

Ten years after picking up that yoga DVD, I'm still in recovery. After two years of a dedicated yoga and meditation practice along with some other health and lifestyle changes I made, I stopped having regressions. I was able to do more and more with my day without worrying that I'd pay for it later. My pain lessened, and the fatigue began to lift.

Yoga and meditation led me to a new way of thinking about my body and about what the words *illness* and *health* mean. It gave me the tools I needed to manage my pain and fatigue, and live a full life, even when I wasn't feeling my best. Eventually, it led to my full recovery.

I wondered why doctors weren't recommending yoga and meditation to patients with chronic fatigue and fibromyalgia. Was I an anomaly? I started researching to see if I could find anyone else who had found recovery through yoga and if there was any science to back it up. The findings were astounding. The research was new, but it was showing that yoga and meditation were helpful for many chronic conditions and diseases. I also found other personal stories of people who had found full or partial recovery through yoga. Over the 10 years since I've been practising, yoga is slowly making its way into mainstream medical advice.

As I prepared to write this book, the studies I found left me in awe of the power of the body-mind/mind-body connection. Western medicine is an incredible tool and has helped cure many illnesses that used to lead to death or disability. Yet, the way that western medicine breaks the body into parts or diseases into symptoms often overlooks a big part of the way our bodies function. While this outlook can be helpful for acute illnesses, in the case of a chronic condition like Fibromyalgia, it's leaving a lot of people without proper treatment.

I don't think we need to do away with western medical practices. Eastern and western medicinal traditions complement each other, and we should use them together. Universal healing strategies like deep breathing, yoga, diet, etc. can be used in conjunction with specific healing strategies like the right medication or surgery. I prefer to use the word complementary medicine rather than alternative medicine because we don't need to choose one or the other. We should use all the tools we have to promote healing.

I mentioned that yoga and mindfulness didn't only change the way I felt, they changed my perspective on life. I realized that I wanted to live a life that helped others, and that was supportive of my health. It was for these reasons I decided to become a yoga teacher, and now, write this book.

I hope this book will help you to understand your pain better, and give you a variety of tools to manage your pain on your journey to recovery.

This book contains seven steps that will help you understand your pain, and practical tips you can use to feel better. The first two steps focus on understanding your pain and cover both the scientific and yogic perspectives on pain management. These chapters help explain why yoga and meditation have been so helpful to so many people. If you're having a brain fog kind of day, you might not take everything in from these chapters, but that's okay. The next five steps focus on practical things you can try, and they are the most crucial part of the book. As Pattabhi Jois, the found of Ashtanga yoga, says:

"Yoga is 1% theory and 99% practice"

As a special thank you for picking up this book, you can download a free copy of the Chronic Pain Workbook, which will help you work through each section of this book and find the practices that work best for you!

To claim your free copy, visit arogayoga.com/chronic-pain-journal/

If you're ready to get started with a deeper understanding of how yoga and mindfulness can help with your pain, read on!

Sending light and love,

Kayla

Step One: Understanding Your Pain

Pain is a neural signal from your body to your brain (and sometimes from your brain to your body) telling you that something is wrong. Pain can be acute or chronic and can feel sharp, dull, throbbing, or ever-present. It can be a small amount of pain like a dull ache, or it can be debilitating pain that keeps you from participating in or enjoying your daily life.

Acute pain is short-lived, and usually a sign you've injured yourself in some way, for example, stubbing your toe or breaking an arm. Chronic pain is more complex and can have a variety of causes. Chronic pain can be in one or several areas of the body, but it's most common in the joints, lower back, shoulders, neck, and head. Sometimes, illness or lifestyle choices (e.g. Bad posture) can cause pain. However, pain does not always have a known cause.

Chronic pain can be something present all the time such as in Arthritis and Fibromyalgia. It can also be intermittent but constant pain such as migraine headaches.

While feeling pain can be worrisome, it isn't necessarily harmful. It is your body's way of communicating with the brain and pain can be there to protect you from further injuring yourself, or letting a severe illness go untreated. Of course, feeling pain all the time when you don't know the cause can be very stressful.

We used to have a simplistic understanding of pain - that it signalled the brain as a direct result of a physical stimulus. Yet, further research on pain is proving that this is not always true. In many cases, there is no physical damage present, but the patient can still be experiencing intense pain.

Pain, no matter the cause, makes your *fight or flight* response go off. When the pain is acute, this can be a helpful reaction. If you've been attacked and feel pain, you know it's time to run away. If you've put your hand too close to a burning flame, you know not to do it again.

However, when it comes to chronic pain, if your *fight or flight* response (known as the sympathetic nervous system) is always on high alert, this can cause you more pain and make it harder to heal.

The fight or flight response is part of the autonomic nervous system (ANS). Within the ANS there's the sympathetic (*fight or flight*) system and the parasympathetic (*rest and digest*) system.

The fight or flight response is a normal and healthy response to some situations. If there's a bear behind us, we want our sympathetic nervous system to activate. Yet, it becomes a dysfunction when it turns on for fibromyalgia pain that is constant, instead of giving the body a chance to rest and heal.

When the sympathetic nervous system is activated, you'll notice that:

- Your heart rate increases
- Your muscles tense
- Digestion slows down
- Your breath becomes shallow

- Your palms begin to sweat

If you've ever gotten butterflies in your stomach before doing something you were nervous about, you've experienced the effects of the sympathetic nervous system. If you're living with fibromyalgia, you may even feel as though you experience those things on a daily basis.

When the parasympathetic nervous system is activated, you'll notice that:

- Digestion improves
- Your muscles relax
- Your heart rate slows down
- You can breathe deeper

Which one of these symptoms would you guess promotes better healing for chronic pain? I think we can all agree it's the second one. The parasympathetic nervous system creates the space that the body needs to heal and relax. Treating the symptoms of pain by taking painkillers or getting a massage won't have any lasting effect if we can't learn to activate the parasympathetic nervous system and keep our muscles relaxed after the effects of the medication or treatment wear off.

The yogic view on suffering is somewhat different than the traditional scientific view of pain. However, recent research on pain is starting to line up closer to the yogic idea of a mind-body connection.

As we said, pain is the way your body communicates danger to your brain. Yet, this danger may not always be a physical sensation, even if your brain perceives it that way. Let's take a look at an example:

Your child is playing outside, and trips on the curb, scraping her knee on the pavement. She starts to cry, and runs inside for you to 'fix it'. A few days later, your child is playing outside on the grass. She trips and falls, but this time she is met by soft ground rather than the pavement. What does your child do? She may get up and continue playing. She may begin crying again, even if there is no scrape this time. What you'll notice is, she'll pause for a moment. She knows what's supposed to happen when you fall over. It's supposed to hurt. This may cause her to start crying, thinking she's hurt. Or it may cause her to take a moment to register a new experience – it doesn't hurt to fall on the grass. If she does begin crying, does that mean she's a crybaby and not experiencing any real pain? Of course not. We already know that pain is viewed as signals the body sends to the brain. But it can sometimes work the other way around too. If your child's brain thinks falling is supposed to hurt, it may send pain signals to the body even if there is no physical damage.

Pain is not as straightforward as we once imagined. The way your body experiences pain depends on your expectations, experiences, and emotions at the time. It can depend on whether help (mom) is nearby or not. It only takes a moment for your brain to process all these things, so it is a process not many of us are aware of. Once your brain has processed this information, it will decide on how high the sensation of pain should be to communicate to your conscious brain how much danger it thinks you're in.

In the yogic world, the mind and body are irrevocably connected. If you find this model of pain trickier to understand, let's look at another example, going back to our *fight or flight* response:

Let's say you're being chased in the woods by a wolf. As you're running, you trip and scrape your knee. In fact, you've tripped on the exact same root you did last week when you went for a run in the woods. That time, you went back to home to patch it up because it was too painful to continue running. However, this time, your brain decides that this pain is not as great as the pain that awaits you if you stop running. You probably won't feel any pain in your knee until your brain is convinced you are out of immediate danger. Once that happens, your brain will start to want you to pay attention to more minor threats, like a scraped or bruised knee.

This is an example to show you that pain is not always consistent. Even when living with chronic pain, the pain may ebb and flow depending on what else is going on in your life. It may depend on how well you slept last night, the weather, work or life stress, etc.

Many sufferers of fibromyalgia will be left without help because their doctors can't find a physical cause to their pain. However, the pain they're feeling in their bodies is genuine, despite lack of physical evidence for it. I remember when I studied psychology in university, we learned about amputees who can still feel sensation in limbs they've had amputated[1]. Up to 80% of amputees feel sensations in a limb that is no longer there, and most of these sensations are pain. This shows how little we know about how the body experiences pain. If you're living with fibromyalgia, you may be frustrated if people think you're faking it or exaggerating because no one can find a physical cause for your pain. Yet, if we look at pain research, this is not something unique to fibromyalgia. There have been several theories of what causes phantom limb pain, but scientists still aren't sure exactly what causes the pain.

Another example of how pain is not always physical is called sympathetic pain[2]. Up to 25% of people experience sympathetic pain, which is the term applied to people who experience pain when they see others in pain. This is especially true for parents who see their children in pain. Yet, even people watching the news or hearing stories of violence can experience sympathetic pain. I mention these theories to show that just because you are experiencing an intense physical sensation of pain, it doesn't mean the cause is physical. It can be a combination of a number of things that are a part of your environment. Yet, it in no way implies that the pain you're experiencing isn't a real, physical sensation.

Understanding that you may be able to treat pain not by treating a physical cause, but by addressing the environment that creates the pain (such as stress, thought patterns, sleeping habits, beliefs, etc.) is a massive breakthrough in the world of pain research. More than that, it starts to explain why so many people find yoga, meditation, and mindfulness a useful tool for managing chronic pain. Yoga sees the body and mind as connected. It's a two-way street.

The western world often takes a specific approach to pain. Rather than looking at the whole person and trying to create balance, it tries to pinpoint the pain and either remove the cause or dull the symptoms. This approach can be beneficial in cases of acute pain. If you break your arm, you should go to the doctor and have the specific symptom (broken arm) treated. No matter how much yoga or meditation you do, you won't stop the pain until you've fixed the cause.

But sometimes this approach isn't so practical. I remember once my doctor advised me to not run if I felt knee pain when running. A holistic approach would be to refer me to a physical therapist who might be able to correct my running stride or a muscular imbalance in my legs. It also went wrong for me when I went from sleeping pill to sleeping pill to sleeping pill, desperate to find a good night's sleep. But the pills weren't helping me get to the root of the problem, which was hyper-arousal before bed. Medication can provide a temporary fix by forcing me to relax. But as soon as I built up a tolerance for the pills, there was my insomnia again. It wasn't until I learned how to deeply relax that I was able to sleep through the night.

Western medicine isn't equipped to deal with non-life threatening chronic conditions. Things like chronic pain or fatigue or insomnia are complicated issues. They don't often get priority in medical research because they aren't causing imminent danger.

This is why many people with chronic illnesses seek complementary medicine.

All that said the scientific world is starting to take an interest in yoga and meditation. They've heard the stories of people like me who have used it to recover from illness, and are starting to study it. Research in the field is new but looks very promising. Many doctors are already beginning to recommend meditation or yoga to their patients living with chronic illnesses.

Action Steps

1) Start a journal or spread sheet to track your progress over the next 2 months. Make a column to measure your pain levels, and start recording times you feel in pain. What happened the night before you had a pain flare? What happened an hour before? How long did it last?

Step Two: Understanding The Science of Yoga

Yoga is more than just a form of exercise. It comes from a medical system called Ayurveda, which is over 2000 years old and originates in ancient India. Ayurveda is often referred to as yoga's sister science and is still practised in India and other places around the world. In India, some Ayurvedic doctors and hospitals have adapted ancient systems to modern times.

Ayurveda takes a holistic approach to healthcare. Rather than treating symptoms, Ayurveda looks at the whole person. It investigates your genetic makeup and emotional patterns, and how this affects your health. This is why, when we look at how yoga can help you manage or recover from fibromyalgia (or any illness) we don't look just at the yoga postures. We also look at your mind, body, breath, and lifestyle.

I found Ayurveda helpful in my recovery process because treating the symptoms (which is what my doctor was recommending) wasn't helping me. Without getting to the root cause of the issue, I was only getting Band-Aid solutions.

My doctors were confused about what chronic fatigue and fibromyalgia were. It's hard to cure something you don't understand. Because Ayurvedic medicine takes a holistic approach to healthcare, they can identify the combination of things such as genetics, bacterial imbalances, emotional blockages or thought patterns, physical ailments, or lifestyle choices that may be causing your illness.

Another reason why I love the Ayurvedic approach to healthcare is that it doesn't put everyone in the same category. In Ayurveda, there are three main dosha's, or dispositions, that we each have. Most people will be dominant in one or two of these dosha's, but, some people are balanced between all three. When one of the dosha's is out of balance, it can cause mild or temporary symptoms, but if the dosha goes unbalanced for too long, it can lead to serious illness.

If you visit an Ayurvedic doctor, the first thing that they'll do is determine your dosha. Instead of looking only at your symptoms, they'll look at your body type, emotional patterns, and genetic dispositions to determine which kinds of foods, events, or lifestyle choices may trigger illness in you. This can vary from person to person. For example, I now know that changing my diet (by removing gluten, dairy, and anything breaded or deep fried) made me feel a lot better. But a lot of my friends eat grilled cheese sandwiches and fish and chips and feel fine. It doesn't mean that there's anything wrong with me, it just means we have different dispositions that react differently to the same stimuli.

The three doshas are:

• Kapha: Content and deliberate, Kapha's have a broad, sturdy build, thick hair, smooth skin, and tend to move slowly. Kapha's will be drawn to slow types of movement like yin yoga and enjoy nurturing those around them.

• Pitta: Fiery and intense, Pitta's are quick to anger, and often have a medium build with yellowish or reddish skin and are prone to red hair and freckles. Pitta's are competitive and high achieving so will be drawn to an active yoga practice like Ashtanga.

• Vata: Airy and scattered, Vata's love talking about many ideas and can never seem to get warm. They have a thin build often with knobbly joints. Vata's resist forming a routine, and are drawn to quick movements like a vinyasa class.

Ayurvedic principles hold that when one dosha is out of balance (whatever balance may mean for an individual's constitution), the imbalance can negatively affect the mind or body. If left untreated this can lead to illness. For example, when vata is out of balance, it can cause insomnia, anxiety, running thoughts, dry skin and nails, gas, bloating, brain fog, and a dislike of cold. To many with fibromyalgia, these symptoms will sound all too familiar. Insomnia, problems with memory, and trouble with digestion are all characteristic of fibromyalgia in addition to the pain.

Many things can cause vata to become imbalanced, such as eating foods that are hard for you to digest, lifestyle choices, and emotional trauma. If you are primarily a vata person, any stress can cause the dosha to become imbalanced. Also, keep in mind that stress weakens your immune system. If you went through a stressful period in life, this makes you more susceptible to picking up a virus, which could, in turn, lead to a dosha imbalance and a more severe illness like fibromyalgia.

In Ayurvedic medicine, there is no one size fits all cure. What is recommended to you by an Ayurvedic practitioner will depend on your individual constitution. This is why in yoga, especially when practising yoga from a book or DVD; your body is always your best teacher. If any of the exercises later in this book make you feel worse, please stop immediately, and consult with your healthcare practitioner and a qualified yoga therapist before trying it again.

To balance the vata dosha, Ayurvedic medicine makes a few key recommendations:

1. Meditate to calm the mind
2. Use breath work to observe the energy in your body
3. Practice grounding asana postures to soothe the body
4. Consider your diet
5. Improve your sleep
6. Practice self-care for your mind, body, and soul

In the rest of this book, we'll get into detail with practical tips on how you can do these things. We'll also pull from scientific research to discover where it agrees with Ayurvedic principles and where it does not.

As you move through this book, remember that Ayurveda is an individualistic way of looking at medical treatment. Everything that works for me might not work for you and visa versa. However, we can look at best practices, and draw from what has worked for others. I can't promise you specific results, but I can tell you what has worked for me, and for my students to help us lead full and pain-free lives. I urge you to work your way through this book with an open mind, before deciding if it works or doesn't work for you. Once you've completed the book and given yourself eight weeks to try out these steps, then you can decide which things you want to keep doing (if any) and which you want to drop.

I'm excited to embark on this healing journey with you as we move on to the next step, taming the mind...

Action Steps

1) Take this quiz to find out what your dosha is. Then take this quiz to find out which dosha's are out of balance. [1]

2) Remember to keep an open mind until the end of this book. See if there is anything helpful for you in understanding your dosha.

---

[1] If you're reading the print version of this book, head to

Step Three: Taming the Mind

In my years as a yoga therapist, I cannot count how many people have told me they can't meditate or do yoga because they have a running mind. If you also feel this way, you're not alone. The idea that we should turn off our minds or stop thinking during a yoga or meditation session is one of the most frustrating myths I come up against as a yoga therapist.

There's no way we can force our minds to stop thinking. Even when we sleep, we can't shut off our brains.

The goal of mindfulness is not to turn off your thoughts. The goal is to observe your thoughts as if from a distance. This objective stops you from getting emotionally involved with each idea as it enters your mind. After all, your thoughts are not facts. They're not the truth. They're just thoughts. When we become too invested in our thoughts, just like becoming too invested in your best friend's relationship drama, it can cause a drain on your energy levels and your stress levels to rise. The goal of mindfulness is to keep our stress levels manageable by interacting with our thoughts objectively.

Being mindful means, we are not worrying about the future or dwelling on the past. We might be observing thoughts or anxieties about those things, but our consciousness always stays in the present.

When we can observe our thoughts, we can also expand that awareness to other sensations and events around us. We become present in conversations with loved ones. We notice the sounds of nature or cars zooming past when out for a walk. We Notice the flavours in a dish a friend has prepared. Or we enjoy the smell of freshly baked bread while passing by a bakery.

In mindfulness practice, we withhold judgement on the sensations we are noticing. Our thoughts, the flavours of food, or the smells we're absorbing (even if it's the smell of a diaper that needs to be changed) don't need to be good or bad. We can simply observe their elements without judgement.

Mindfulness doesn't involve trying to change anything. And it certainly doesn't include trying to stop your thoughts. It just means that we are observing what is happening to and around us. Rather than becoming involved in every thought or sensation we experience.

What does the science say about mindfulness?

Thanks to John Kabat-Zinn, the physician who is credited with bringing mindfulness to the western world, the effects on mindfulness meditation on health have been studied more than any other kind of complementary health practice.

In a meta-review (a type of scientific study which reviews a large body of studies done on a subject) done in 2017, it showed that mindfulness did help to decrease pain in chronic pain patients. Specifically symptoms of depression and low quality of life that often go with chronic pain.[3]

Studies have also found that yoga has a more positive effect on health than other forms of exercise such as walking.[4] Doctors have long known that exercise has a positive effect on mood and health. But why does yoga seem to have a stronger effect than other forms of exercise? We don't know for sure, but many in the yoga community believe that it is due to the mindfulness, meditation, and breath work that is used in a yoga practice, as well as the physical postures.

Despite mindfulness being the most researched area in complementary medicine, there is still a long way to go in discovering how mindfulness helps chronic pain sufferers. Due to the variant nature of pain and difficulty in measuring pain consistently from person to person, it can be a hard topic to study. However, many doctors are now recommending meditation to patients who don't respond to traditional treatments.

When it comes to mindfulness, one of the greatest benefits is that there is no harm in trying. While some people I've worked with are hesitant to try yoga because they don't want to make their symptoms worse by overexertion or moving the wrong way, mindfulness doesn't come with any physical risk. You can practice mindfulness on your own, by listening to a recorded meditation track, or by working with a teacher trained in mindfulness meditation.

Primary and Secondary Suffering

Understanding the difference between primary and secondary suffering is essential to understanding how mindfulness can reduce chronic pain.

Primary suffering is the initial pain you experience after physical or emotional trauma. If you stub your toe, for example, that first shot of pain would be primary suffering.

For the most part, we can't help the way primary pain feels. It's caused by something external, and our reaction to it is out of our control, dictated by the subconscious systems of the body.

Secondary suffering is the pain we experience on top of the initial shock. For example, if after stubbing your toe you think to yourself, "Shit! This is the most painful thing that's ever happened to me! I'm sure it's broken!" That is secondary suffering. Most people won't jump to the conclusion that stubbing their toe means it's broken. Yet, when it comes to more serious conditions like relentless chronic pain, it's easy to fall into negative thought patterns. While thoughts like "this pain will never go away", may seem realistic, they can actually make the pain worse.

We now know that the environment we're in (or help create) can affect the amount of pain we feel. So it makes sense that these negative thoughts can make your pain worse without any intention to do so on your part.

An initial adverse reaction to pain is normal. In many situations, it's helpful. It helps your brain process not to do that harmful thing again (e.g. walking without looking where you're going). However, when we don't know the cause of the pain, sustaining these negative thoughts are not helpful.

Stopping these negative thought patterns is easy to talk about, but in practice, it's challenging.

Mindfulness is a tool that we can use to help reprogram the brain and change these thought patterns. In mindfulness, we take a non-judgemental approach to our experiences. This non-judgement helps us differentiate from the pain our mind may be trying to tell us is present, for example, "I always have fibromyalgia and I always feel pain" vs. the pain we are actually experiencing which can change from day to day and moment to moment.

When it comes to using mindfulness to reduce pain, we want to focus on the things we can control. We can choose to practice yoga or meditation; we can decide to monitor our breath; we can take a moment to notice sensations in our body.

Focusing on the things we can control also helps us set up for goals that we can achieve. For example, the goal to lose 10 pounds would not be an effective yogic goal. You can't control whether you'll be able to lose the weight. However, setting a goal to eat seven servings of fruits and vegetables per day, or exercise three times per week, are both goals in which we can, for the most part, control the results.

Let's apply this principle to setting goals or expectations for chronic pain. Instead of thinking I want to try this new program, diet, doctor, etc. and be completely pain-free, you can set a goal to change negative thought patterns or reduce a lifestyle habit that may be contributing to your pain. It doesn't mean you'll be pain-free, but it does mean that you're taking steps to reduce your pain in a way that you can control.

To summarise, secondary pain is the pain that is most affected by us, by our thoughts, feelings, emotions, or lifestyle habits. It's the pain that we can control, and focus on reducing. The primary pain will still be present, but we can reduce the amount of pain we feel by lowering our secondary suffering.

Pain Acceptance

True, deep acceptance opens the path to healing. By accepting the pain present in our body, we can begin to reduce secondary suffering. If you start to become aware of pain at different points throughout the day, you'll begin to see that your pain is not constant. It may feel different at certain times of the day. It may be stronger when you're under stress and slightly less when feeling relaxed. If you pay attention you'll realize your pain is not permanent – it is flowing and ever-changing. While this means your pain could get much worse, it also means your pain can get better. We don't know what will happen, all we do know is that the pain changes. As Heraclitus says: "The only thing that is constant, is change".

Thoughts like "I'll never get better", or "this pain will never go away", or "I'll never be able to have what I want in life", can all seem like realistic ways to grieve – and are perfectly understandable thoughts to have. But, these thought patterns can add to your suffering. You don't know if your pain will go away or not. You don't know if it will get better or worse. All you know is what is happening in your body at the moment. We can't possibly know the outcome in the future, we can only try to accept the present.

When in pain, it's a normal response to want to fight and resist this pain. Phrases like "we can beat this" are common amongst patient groups and charities for illnesses. It feels like we're going to a championship sports match and want to win, not working with our bodies, which we love and cherish. What if the fighting approach, while a natural response, is the wrong way response? What if this is creating more pain rather than eliminating it?

What if instead of "I will beat this pain" we say "I will work with this pain and my body in a respectful way to live my fullest life."

Acceptance of your pain is not resignation. It is simply acknowledging the situation as it is in this moment. It is allowing yourself to stop struggling against yourself and letting peace and kindness take its place. Once you can make this transition, your stress levels, and secondary suffering will begin to diminish.

Stress and Pain

Stress makes pain worse. It's also true that stress exacerbates any illness from the common cold to cancer. The bottom line is: stress is bad for your health. Once you start to become more aware of the flow of your pain, you'll be able to monitor better which activities are stressful and cause your pain to get worse or flare.

Stress combined with pain can create a cycle that is hard to break without mindful intention. You feel pain, which makes you feel stressed out, which makes you feel more pain, which makes you feel even more stressed out!

So how can you break this cycle?

We know that pain is a signal that your body is sending to your brain that something is wrong. This signal activates the sympathetic nervous system. If your pain is acute, or life-threatening, this response is necessary for survival. Your heart rate will increase, your breath will become shallow, your muscles will tense, your pupils will dilate, your palms might sweat, and that feeling of butterflies in your stomach? That's the muscles in your intestines slowing down movement. Your body is programming you to put all of your mental and physical energy towards stopping the threatening situation. When you're living with chronic pain, this response is exhausting.

Yoga and meditation systemically work to deepen your breath and relax your muscles. Researchers have found that yoga and meditation significantly lower levels of cortisol – the hormone in the brain that is associated with stress.

Doing yoga or meditating can have a long-term effect on how we manage stress. Another study found that people who regularly meditate bounce back from stress faster than those who do not have a consistent practice[5]. Let's take a look at this example to see how stress can affect your pain, and the effect that meditation can have on stress:

You're out for a walk and want to cross the street. You're having a flare-up with severe brain fog and accidentally look the wrong way. You hear a car horn and jump out of the way just in time to avoid getting hit by a car. What's happening inside your body at this moment? The stress response is in full swing. Since this was a life-threatening situation, your body is appropriately responding to the risk at hand. Those who don't meditate may carry the stress of that incident with them for the rest of the day. But, those who regularly meditate or practice mindfulness can calm their bodies' down faster and return to normal levels of stress hormones after the upsetting incident.

Just as mindfulness doesn't mean stopping your thoughts, meditating or mindfulness doesn't mean you will always be calm and relaxed and never feel stressed. I feel stressed out all the time! However, if you build a regular mindfulness practice, you'll be able to better manage and overcome that stress. Returning to homeostasis after a stressful event helps keep the nervous system balanced, and can keep your symptoms from worsening under pressure.

Not only can pain itself be stressful, but thinking about pain or triggers for the pain can cause stress. For example, if you often have pain when you wake up in the morning, or after going for a walk, the anticipation and monitoring of that pain can cause even more stress. Being mindful helps us live in the moment, and let go of anticipation stress.

Engaging in activities that help reduce stress on a regular basis such as yoga, meditation and systemic relaxation can help reduce the amount of pain you experience. However, it's not just yoga and meditation that can help reduce stress. Partaking in a hobby you love, reading your favourite book, spending time outside, exercising, spending time with friends and family, and cooking your favourite meal can all help lower your stress levels.

Not all activities that we see as relaxing are indeed relaxing. For example, spending a lot of time in front of a screen, especially at night, can be arousing for the body. Watching movies or TV shows or reading books with a lot of violence or suspense can also stimulate the nervous system and make it hard to sleep.

If you have trouble sleeping, this can exacerbate pain. While we can't control whether we sleep, we can work to create the conditions for a good night's sleep by creating good sleep habits (more on this in step six). We can also build a yoga practice designed to help rest. We'll go over what this could look like in step five.

Mindfulness Practices

Mindfulness meditation focuses on building awareness. This may be awareness of the body, awareness of your thoughts, awareness of the senses, or awareness of the things around you.

Some of the most popular types of mindfulness meditation are:

A Body Scan

A body scan involves moving your attention through different parts of your body and noticing any feelings or sensations present. An important part of the body scan is to suspend judgement over whether these feelings are good or bad. You should simply notice how they feel. For example, is the feeling heavy or light? Tight or loose? Dull or aching? You don't even need to use words to describe your feelings, but just move your awareness to a certain part of your body and pay attention.

How to do it:

- Lie down on a yoga mat or your bed. This can also be done seated in a chair, but I recommend lying down for beginners, as it's not uncommon to fall asleep during the practice! Begin by focusing on your breath, breathing slowly and deeply.
- As you inhale, bring your focus down to your feet, noticing any sensations in your toes, heels, or the top or bottom of the feet. Hold your attention here for 2-3 breaths. On the next exhale release your attention.
- As you inhale again, move the attention up to the ankles and calves.
- Continue moving your attention through the body from your toes to your head, moving your focus every few breaths.
- Suspend passing judgement on the things you notice in your body. Allow any feelings – even pain – to reside in your body.

- Finish the meditation by bringing your awareness to your entire body at once, and then slowly moving the fingers and the toes before sitting up.

Breathing Meditation

As you can guess from the name, this meditation focuses on your breath. You can visualize your breath moving in and out of the body and through the respiratory system, you can focus on physical sensations of the breathing, or count your breath to stay focused.

How to do it:

- Lie down or sit in a comfortable position free from distractions or interruptions.
- Begin by focusing on your breath. Notice how the breath feels moving in and out of your nostrils, all the way down into your diaphragm.
- Picture the breath moving in through your nose, down the back of your throat, through your lungs, and down into your belly. Imagine you can see the breath re-tracing this routes back out into the room.
- After 5-10 rounds of visualizing your breath, count your breaths up to 10, then back down to one, counting each breath on the exhale.
- Once you've come back to one, take a few more breaths, noticing how your body feels, and then open your eyes.

Thought Observation

I mentioned earlier in this chapter that one of the pillars of mindfulness is observing your thoughts. This meditation helps you to actively observe your thoughts without becoming attached to them. This meditation can help reduce anxiety or overthinking. Thoughts are not facts or morsels of truth. They simply come and go as we inhale and exhale.

How to do it:

- Sit in a comfortable position free from distractions or interruptions, and start with a short breathing meditation.
- Slowly begin to shift your focus from your breath to your thoughts.
- Acknowledge the thoughts running through your mind and allow them to stay there, while still being aware of your breath, and what is happening in the present moment. I sometimes find it helpful to repeat my thoughts in my head by saying to myself "I'm thinking about what I want for dinner now, okay. I'm thinking about that really embarrassing moment where I fell in front of my co-workers earlier today okay that's fine, but right now I'm doing a meditation and am breathing, and am sitting, and am noticing."
- If you find yourself responding emotionally to your thoughts, or you spiral into a thought train, it can help to listen to a guided meditation so you have someone to remind you to come back to the

present. This can be a difficult meditation, especially for those of us with a mind that easily wanders, but it can also be one of the most rewarding in reducing stress and anxiety.

- After 10-15 minutes bring your focus back to your breath to come out of the meditation.

Expanding Awareness

This meditation includes elements of the above three meditations. You'll begin by focusing on your breath and then reach out through all five senses until your have complete awareness of your body and surroundings. This is an advanced type of mindfulness meditation.

How to do it:

- Sit or lie in a comfortable position free from distractions.
- Start with a breathing meditation.
- Move into a body scan meditation.
- Move into a thought observation meditation.
- Begin to bring your senses into awareness. What can you hear? Feel? Smell?
- Bring any people or pets in the area into your awareness.
- See if you can hold all of these things, both inside of you and outside of you in your awareness at once.
- Return to focusing on your breath or a breathing meditation.

- Finish the meditation with a few slow breaths, and open your eyes.

Moving Meditation

When yoga originated, the physical postures were created to help monks stay physically healthy while sitting in meditation for long periods of time. One of my first yoga teachers told me that yoga was a moving meditation, and I've always kept that thought with me when I'm doing my physical yoga practice. However, a moving meditation isn't limited to yoga. It can be other forms of exercise like tai chi, chi gong, or even going for a slow walk while noticing how your body feels and your surroundings.

How to do it:

- Choose which activity you'd like to do mindfully. If it's yoga, you can follow some of the sequences later in this book, so for the purposes of this chapter, we'll cover a walking meditation.
- Find a place to walk that isn't too busy. You can do this inside your house, in a park, or on a quiet street. It's hard to stay focused in a meditation if you have to keep looking out for people or cars!
- Begin by standing, and doing a mini expanding meditation, first by focusing on your breath, and then your body.
- As you start to walk, notice how your body feels when moving. Notice how it feels on your feet to

make contact with the ground. Notice which muscles you're using and how your body moves.

- If you find your mind starts to wander, it can be helpful to count your steps.
- Do this meditation for as long as you find it comfortable.

If you're new to meditation, I recommend starting with the body scan and breathing meditation. As you get more comfortable you can move onto the thought observation and expanding awareness meditations. Moving meditation is something that you can practice every day, either during your yoga practice, walking around your house, or going out for a walk in nature. We'll talk more about incorporating mindfulness into your daily life in the last chapter of this book.

Action Steps

1) Set a mindful goal for your pain management plan. What can you commit to doing where you will have control over the results? Write this goal down and stick it up somewhere in your house where you will see it every day. Also add this goal to your tracking sheet from step one.

2) Choose one of the mindfulness practices mentioned in this chapter and practice it for 10 minutes, three times this week. Record how you feel before and after in a journal.

Step Four: Using the Breath as an Energy Source

While mindfulness focuses on observing and giving attention to the breath, pranayama focuses on controlling the breath.

Pranayama is the yogic word for breath control or breathing exercises. Prana is the Sanskrit word for breath or life force. Ayama means to restrain or control. These exercises are intended to clear any blocks you have so that the prana can flow freely through you. The concept of prana is similar to the idea of chi in traditional Chinese medicine.

If you go to a yoga class in a gym or a yoga studio focused on fitness, the amount of meditation and breathing exercises in the class may be limited. However, if you are working with a yoga therapist, meditation and breath work will become an essential part of your yoga practice.

One thing I love about breath work and meditation in the treatment of chronic pain is that, just like mindful meditation, you can do them every day. Even on days when you feel in too much pain or too tired to do a physical yoga practice or even get out of bed, you can still do a breathing exercise.

In the body, we have voluntary and involuntary actions. Voluntary actions are things we do consciously, such as walking, talking, eating, etc. Involuntary actions are things that happen automatically such as your heart beating, digestion of food, etc. Breathing is an involuntary activity – if you try to stop breathing, you'll pass out, and your body will automatically start breathing for you. Yet, we can also control our breath to some extent. We can hold our breath, breathe deeply, breathe shallowly, through the nose, through the mouth, noisily, quietly, etc. It's because of this reason that yogi's see pranayama as an essential daily routine. It connects both the voluntary and involuntary systems.

Because breathing is the only involuntary system we can control, breathing practices can be a powerful tool to uncouple other automatic associations we make. For example, your negative emotions or pain can become part of your identity. Sometimes, we subconsciously hold on to suffering because we see it as a part of who we are. You may also associate certain triggers or actions with pain, and breaking these associations can help reduce pain. You can't completely break these associations, but we can reduce it, so you don't feel as overwhelmed by the pain.

When I started practising yoga, I only practised mindfulness meditations. As I learned more about pranayama, I began incorporating these breathing exercises into my daily practice. I used to have a chronically stuffed nose and struggled to breathe nasally. When I started practising yogic breathing exercises my sinuses cleared up, and for the first time that I could remember, I was able to breathe through my nose!

I recommend practising both pranayama and mindfulness or other forms of meditation. Pranayama can help prepare the mind for meditation and can help you get into a deeper meditative state thus increasing the health benefits of meditation. Pranayama can also be a meditation on its' own.

Breathing is a thing you do all day, every day. But it can be a powerful tool for improving your health by paying attention to it or controlling it. Diaphragmatic breathing (breathing deeply into your diaphragm, so your belly rises on each inhalation) is refreshing and restful and creates a sense of wellbeing. Because we are always breathing, breath awareness is a self-management tool that is useful even during the busiest times of the day.

What does the science say about Pranayama?

While the effects of a specific kind of pranayama have not been studied, there is some research to indicate that breathing through your nose, and diaphragmatic breathing, both reduce stress and activate the parasympathetic nervous system. Two studies have found that pranayama reduced heart rate and blood pressure after practicing for just 15 days![6]

Here are some of my favourite pranayama exercises:

Alternate nostril breathing

While alternate nostril breathing was recently made famous by Hilary Clinton (when asked how she coped with the election loss, she responded by demonstrated alternate nostril breathing), yogi's have been practicing this breathing technique for hundreds of years.

This breathing exercise is also the most effective in giving me *yoga brain* – what yoga practitioners refer to as the feeling of being both relaxed and alert. This exercise can give you a burst of energy, help you feel calm, and enhance your mental functioning.

How to do it:

- Sit in a comfortable position on a chair or the floor.
- Place your left hand on your knee. With your right hand, extend the thumb and ring finger.
- Place the thumb just over your right nostril, and your ring finger just over the left.
- To begin, close the left nostril with your finger, and inhale through the right. Hold the breath while you release the left nostril and cover the right. Exhale through the left nostril.
- On your next inhale breathe through the left nostril. Hold the breath as you switch fingers, and exhale through the right.
- Continue for 3-5 minutes.

Bee breath

Many people find the bee breath (officially known as brahmari) helps with anxiety. Since chronic pain can cause feelings of anxiety, I find it a helpful practice – particularly before bed or anytime you're feeling stressed. As the name implies, this exercise requires making a buzzing noise as you breathe out.

How to do it:

- Sit in a comfortable position on the floor or in a chair. Begin breathing through the nose.
- After your next inhale, make an extended MMMMM sound as you exhale, just as the last syllable in the OM chant. When you are all out of breath to exhale, inhale, and repeat.

Yoga Nidra

Yoga nidra, or yogic sleep, is a meditation practice that helps you cultivate a sense of safety and wellbeing. It is best practiced after doing pranayama.

I was several years into my yoga practice before I tried yoga nidra. I was sceptical because I had found so much relief from mindfulness meditation. Why should I learn something new if I already had something that was working well? But now, not only do I love my yoga nidra practice, I can see the way that it helps my students, especially those who have trouble with pain. If you have severe chronic pain, you may find it hard to concentrate in a mindfulness meditation because the pain is too intense. However, yoga nidra takes us out of our bodies and cultivates a space away from the stress and pain.

A yoga nidra session of 30-60 minutes can sometimes have the same benefits to the body that sleep has. So, if you struggle with getting enough high-quality sleep, this is definitely a tool you should add to your basket.

Yoga nidra uses guided visualization and imagery to help students get into a deep meditation. At the beginning of the session, you'll create your own oasis, a place you can visualize in your mind where you feel completely safe and at ease. Then, drawing on these feelings, we can continue through the guided meditation.

Since yoga nidra is a guided meditation, it's not something you can practice on your own. You'll need a recording to help you, or will need to join a yoga nidra class or session in public.

In contrast to mindfulness meditation where we aim to observe, not interact, with our thoughts, in yoga nidra, we welcome thoughts and feelings during the practice. While we still don't judge these thoughts or feelings, we can actively aim to balance them. For example, if you're feeling stress or anxiety, you can cultivate feelings of calmness.

Yoga nidra has recently become popular for people with anxiety and PTSD, and many programs have arisen to help veterans. I think that this can also be a very helpful practice for those with chronic pain who need a respite from the sensations in their body.

Action Steps

1) Try out each of the pranayama practices. Write down how you feel both before and after doing the practice.

Step Five: Yoga Postures to Relieve Pain

A quick note before starting this chapter: you should speak with your doctor before starting any new physical activity plan. Your doctor can help you identify any potential challenging movements that you'll want to discuss with your yoga therapist, or be aware of when starting a home practice. The first rule of yoga is that we don't want to make anything worse. If you have bad knees, high or low blood pressure, or anything else that may affect your yoga practice, you should talk with your doctor to discuss if there are any postures you should avoid, or adapt, in your yoga practice. If you work with a qualified yoga therapist, they will be able to help you adapt the poses based on your doctor's recommendations.

In this chapter, we'll cover two yoga practices – one for the morning and one for the evening. You're welcome to practice these on the same day, or on alternate days. If you're short on time or energy, you can also select one or two postures to do, even if they are postures you do from bed.

Deciding when, and how often, to practice yoga is up to the individual. Traditionally, yoga is practised in the morning. However, the best practice is the one that we can stick to so I encourage you to find a practice schedule that works for you.

Your yoga practice does not need to last for an hour or more. Even 10 minutes of yoga a day can help you get the benefits of a yoga practice. Studies have shown that people who practice yoga for 10 minutes a day at least five days a week have better results than people who do an hour-long practice only once a week[7].

Yoga and meditation help rewire the brain. In yoga, we call this samaskara, and in the scientific world, it's called neuroplasticity. By creating a new habit, we change our brain. Frequent practices are the most helpful for making these brain changes, even if the duration is short. You don't need to practice every day if that is not possible for you, but aiming to consistently practice three to five times a week for 10-30 minutes a day can change your brain.

We need to move the body in all different directions to keep it healthy. In many forms of exercise, such as walking, we're only moving the body in one direction – front to back. In yoga, we move front to back, side to side, and twist, so that the body can explore its full range of movement. More than just the physical, we'll aim to balance the autonomic nervous system in this practice, combining poses that are both calming and challenging.

Morning Practice

For our morning practice, we'll aim to relieve the stiffness of sleep and warm up the body for the day.

If you struggle to get up in the morning, it can be helpful to lie out the yoga mat in the bedroom or living room floor before going to bed. You can even begin this practice in bed, and then move on to the mat after the first two postures.

1. Start lying down on your back in Savasana (corpse pose). Let your feet fall open to either side and lie with your palms facing up. Begin to focus on your breath, aiming to take long, even, breaths through the nose. Breathing through the nose is ideal for deep yogic breathing, but if you're not able to breathe comfortably through your nose, breathe through the mouth.

If you feel yourself drifting off to sleep, it can be helpful to keep your eyes open in this posture.

After 5-7 rounds of deep breathing, begin to move the arms. On the inhale, move your arms straight up parallel to the body, like zombie's arms. On the exhale, lower them back down to your side. After 2-3 rounds, inhale your arms completely overhead, stretching them out behind you, and exhale lower them back down. Repeat two to three times.

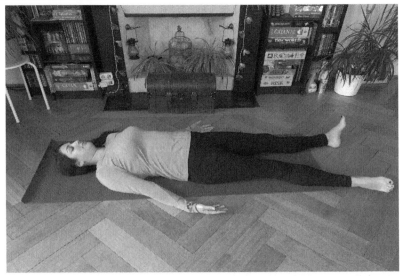

2. Bring your arms back down, and bend your knees, drawing them into your chest. Wrap your arms around your legs, like you're giving yourself a hug. You can stay still here, or rock from side to side to massage the lower back.

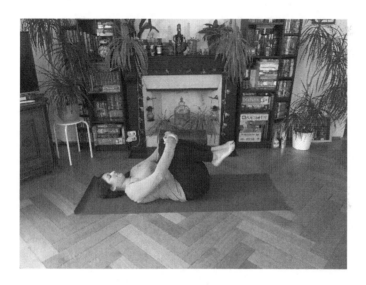

2a. Release the left leg down, and pull the right leg towards the right shoulder. Hold for 20-30 seconds and then release and switch sides. Then, bring both knees back into your chest and roll onto your side.

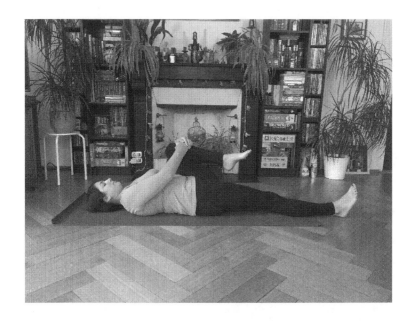

3. From your side, roll all the way onto your hands and knees. Take a couple breaths here to adjust to being upright.

As you inhale, lift your head, open your chest, curve your spine and lift your hips. As you exhale, drop the hips down, round the spine, and let the head hang loose. Repeat for five to seven rounds, using your own breath as a guide for how quickly you move. Allow the spine to move fluidly back and forth from cat to cow like a cooked piece of spaghetti.

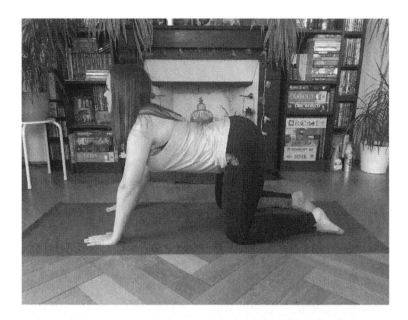

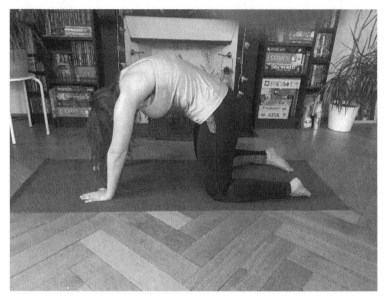

4. Come back to a neutral spine, and then walk your hands forward until your forehead comes down either to

the mat or close to the mat. Keep your hips over your knees, and enjoy a stretch in the upper back and shoulders. Hold for five breaths.

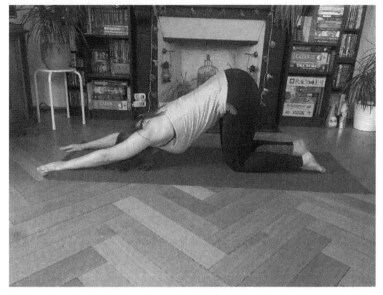

5. Walk the hands back slightly, and curl the toes under. Lift the knees off the mat and stretch the hips towards the ceiling to come into downward facing dog, keeping the knees bent. Hold for five breaths. Then, walk the hands back towards the feet and slowly roll up to a standing position. Stand in Tadasana, mountain pose, with the arms by your side and head reaching tall for five breaths.

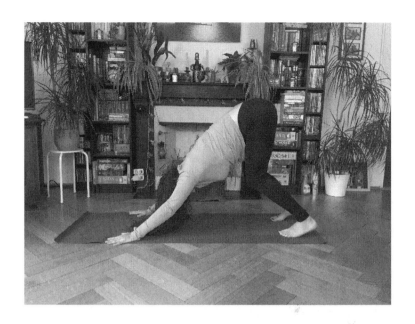

6. Step the left foot back, moving it perpendicular to the mat. The right foot faces forwards. As you inhale, stand up tall and engage the core muscles. Raise your hands straight out to either side. Then, hinge the torso towards the right foot, turning your right hand to your right shin or ankle, and your left arm reaches directly up to the ceiling. Hold for five breaths.

To come out of the pose, look down towards the right foot, and on the inhale, use the strength of the core to come up to centre. Pivot the feet to repeat on the opposite side.

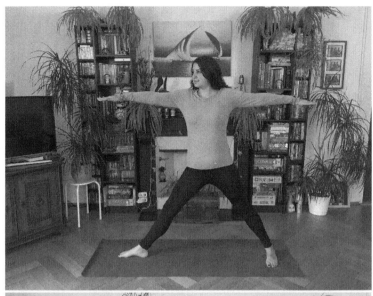

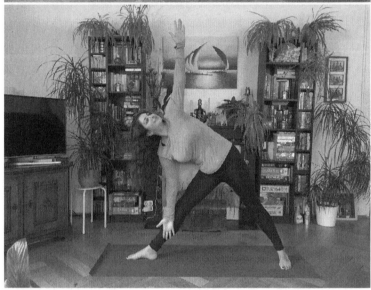

7. Step the feet together at the front of the mat. Take a breath to re-centre before moving to the next pose. Step the left foot back again, placing it at a 90-degree angle.

The right foot faces forwards. Place your hands on your hips to shift the hips forward. If the hips don't move, you can widen your stance by moving your right foot to the right side of the mat. Inhale lengthen the spine, exhale, bend the front knee, coming into a high lunge. You can either keep your hands on your hips or extend the arms up, coming into a micro backbend. Hold for five breaths. To come out of the pose, lower the arms, and step the feet together at the front of the mat. Switch sides.

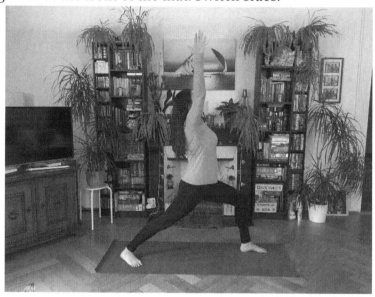

8. Sit down in a comfortable cross-legged position, placing your hands on your knees. If you find it difficult to keep your spine straight in this position, sit on a cushion or chair with your feet on the floor. Inhale to lengthen the spine and sit up tall, as you exhale, move the right hand to the left knee, and place the left hand behind your hips and look over your shoulder. On every inhale

lengthening the spine, and on every exhale twist. Hold for 5-10 breaths, and then switch sides.

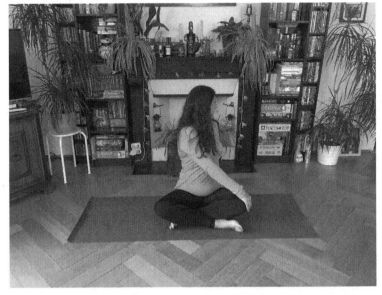

9. Come forward to lie down on your stomach. Slide the forearms in front of you, so that your elbows are beneath your shoulders. If you find this pinches the lower back, slide your arms forwards so that your elbows are slightly in front of the shoulders. Keep the spine neutral and gaze forwards. Hold for 10-15 breaths.

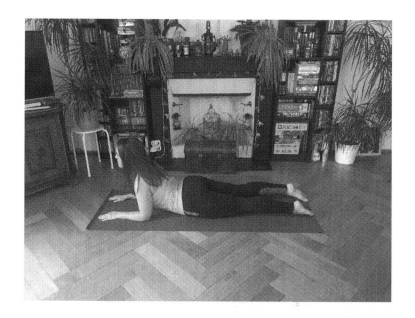

10. Press back on your hands and knees and come all the way back into child's pose. There are two variations of this pose.

10a. Spread your knees as wide as the mat with your feet together. Sit your hips back until your hips reach your heals. If they don't reach, place a cushion or blanket on top of the feet to rest on. Then, walk your hands forward until your forehead reaches the mat. Again, if your forehead does not reach, use a pillow or blanket to support your head and neck.

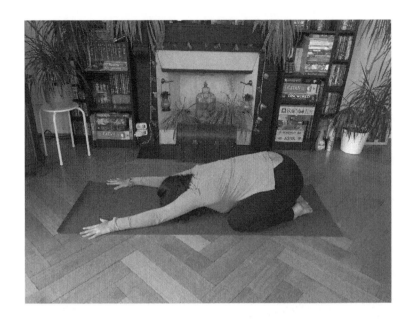

10b. Keep your knees together and sit back on your heels, using a blanket or pillow if your hips are hanging. Then lower your forehead down to the mat, and place your hands with the palms facing up by your hips.

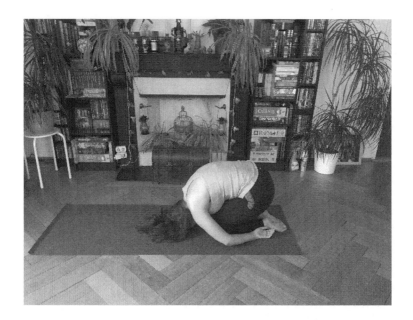

Whichever version of this pose you choose, hold for 10-20 seconds.

End the practice either with a seated meditation or returning to Savasana for several minutes.

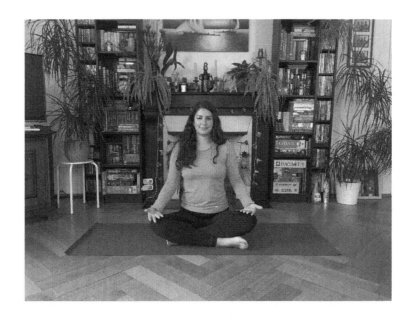

You don't need to do all 10 of these postures every morning, but use these ideas to get into the habit of a short, and regular, morning yoga practice!

Evening Practice

In this evening sequence, we'll focus on releasing tension in the body and relaxing the mind. This is a great yoga practice to do in the evening or before bed. It can also be done in the morning or during the day if you're feeling low on energy.

Because these postures are held for longer periods of time, many people sometimes find them more challenging than a flowing practice. If you experience any pain or discomfort in any of these postures you should come out of the pose and move on to the next one. If you are able to work with a yoga therapist, they'll be able to help you find an alternative that works for you. However, always remember that you are your own best teacher. You know your body better than anyone else.

If you find that your mind is wandering in these postures, first know that you're not alone. Everyone experiences wandering mind syndrome when meditating or doing yoga. If you do find your mind wandering, acknowledge your thoughts, and then make the choice to bring your focus back to your breathing, letting the thoughts flitter in the back of your mind. It can also be helpful to do some of the breathing exercises or meditations we've covered while holding these poses.

For this practice, you'll need a couple of pillows or cushions and a blanket. If you have yoga blocks, those can also be helpful in this practice.

1. Begin in a supported child's pose. Keep your knees separated with your feet together. Take one of your pillows, and slide it between your knees. Then walk your hands forward, resting your right ear down on the pillow. If the position feels strained, you can use a second pillow.

Hold the pose for 2-5 minutes, and then move your head to the other side for another 2-5 minutes.

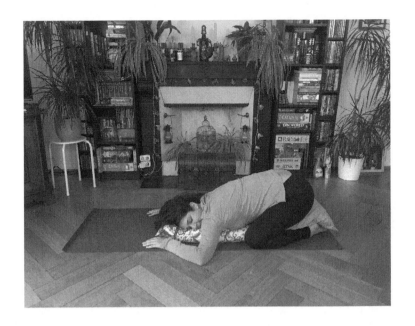

2. Walk your hands up, and come into a normal cross-legged position in front of a chair. Place your hands on the chair, and then rest your head on the chair.

2a. You can have your legs in any position for this posture. If you'd like to change up the stretch try butterfly (badha konasana) or forward leg bend.

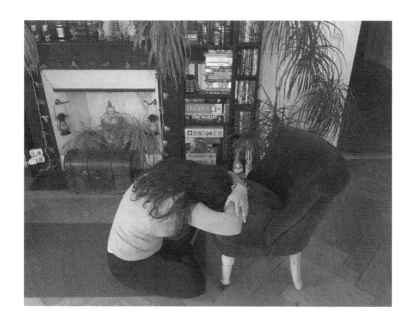

Hold this pose for 3-4 minutes, breathing deeply, and keeping your eyes closed.

3. Slowly come up from this posture, staying in front of the chair. Sitting parallel to the chair (or a wall), place a pillow or cushion behind your hips. Lean back on the cushion and swing your legs up on the wall or chair. Place your left hand on your stomach and your right hand on your heart, feeling the breath moving through your torso.

Hold this posture for three to five minutes.

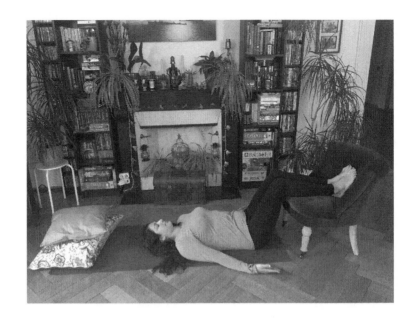

4. Swing your legs off the wall or chair, and move back to your mat for supine butterfly pose. Lie on your back, and bring the soles of the feet together. Experiment with sliding your feet backwards and forwards until you find the ideal place for your feet to rest.

4a. To make this pose more comfortable, you can place pillows, cushions, or blankets under your knees to support the legs and hips. Some people also find bringing a pillow on your belly or chest can add weight to the pose making it more relaxing.

Hold this posture for three to five minutes.

5. To come into your final savasana, stretch your legs out, letting your feet fall to the side, and place your arms by your side with your palms facing up. You might want to place a pillow over your chest under your knees to get very comfortable in this posture.

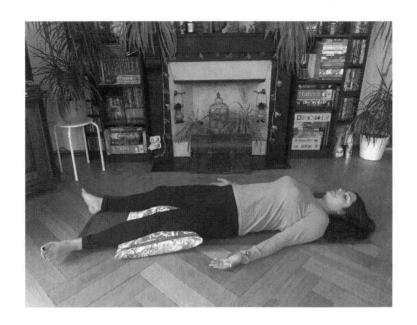

Hold for 5-10 minutes.

You can do these postures before bed or if you wake up during the night and can't fall back asleep. This can help you get back to sleep, or find a place of deep relaxation.

For more 10-15 minute sequences, and to target specific parts of the body such as neck and shoulders, lower back, hips, and hamstrings, check out my 10-day yoga for chronic pain <u>bundle here, or if you have the print version of this book head to www.arogayoga.com and look under the 'online courses' tab.</u>

Yoga During Flare-Ups

A lot of students I've worked with report feeling better after doing yoga for several weeks, but then have a flare-up, and their practice falls away. Once we lose a habit, it's hard to build it up again. Especially if you're in pain.

The good news is some yogic practices can help you get through a flare. You'll just need to adapt your routine to what your body needs. Checking in with your body is a good exercise to do every day, anyways. What you could do yesterday (or five years ago) may be very different than what you can do today.

In yoga, we aim to have a beginner's mind. When we first begin to learn something new, we're open to many possibilities. Because we don't have preconceived notions of what the right way to do a new thing is, we can often see many different paths.

As Zen teacher, Suzuki Roshi said, "In the beginner's mind there are many possibilities, but in the expert's there are few."

Because yoga is becoming more popular, many people start yoga with preconceptions, making it harder to keep a beginner's mind during your practice. This leads many people to feel like they're not good at yoga. We see images of yogi's that are mostly thin, young, flexible, healthy, white women. The reality is there are many different kinds of yoga, yogi's, and yoga practices.

When we remember there is no right way to do yoga it makes planning for flare-ups easier. Yoga is much more than a physical practice, and using meditation and breathing exercises, can help you find ways to maintain your practice during a flare-up.

The first step in maintaining your practice during a flare-up is to have a flare-up plan. When you have a flare-up, doing necessary things like showering or making food can be a struggle, understandably, yoga often falls by the wayside during these times. However, making a plan now, to commit to a non-physical practice during a flare-up can help you keep your practice up during harder times.

Another helpful tip is to find practices that you can do in bed. This can be a mindfulness meditation, yoga nidra, pranayama, visualization, or even a restorative yoga practice.

If you listen to a yoga video and visualize doing the actions without actually moving your body, your muscles can still benefit from this. One study found that people who imagined doing a physical practice got up to 70% of the muscular benefits they would get by actually doing the physical practice! [8]

If you would like to include a physical practice in your flare-up plan, stick to a restorative practice, like the evening sequence in this chapter. You can even pick just one posture from this book to do every day during a flare-up.

I once had a teacher who said, "the intention to practice yoga, is yoga". Remember that yogic goal setting is what we can control, not the outcome. You don't need to do a hard physical practice every day. In fact, if you're having a bad day, you shouldn't aim to do that. You should set a goal to do what is nourishing for your body each day.

Action Steps

1) Set a goal for your yoga practice. How many times a week do you think you can practice? What time of day is best for you?

2) Do it! Set aside the time in your daily calendar to commit to this yoga practice for at least eight weeks.

3) Make a plan for flare-ups. What yoga, breathing, or meditation practices can you do when you're not up for an active yoga practice?

Step Six: Self-Care

Yoga and meditation are great tools for reducing pain and improving your health. There are also other yogic lifestyle changes you can make to complement your yoga practice.

Self-care is a broad term and is used to refer to a variety of activities. In this book, I'm looking at self-care from a yogic perspective. What are other yogic things that we can do to improve our health and nourish our bodies?

From an Ayurvedic perspective, chronic pain is an imbalance of the vata dosha. The recommendations in this chapter will help you to balance the vata dosha by creating routines, and finding slow, nourishing activities that counterbalance the flightiness of vata.

Creating a Morning Routine

Creating a routine is an integral part of the yogic lifestyle. When I lived in an Ashram in India, the wake-up bell rang promptly at 4am every day. We then went to a chanting session, to a chai (tea) session, to a meditation session, and then free time where you could practice yoga or use your neti pot[2]. It wasn't until 8am, four hours after waking up, that we ate breakfast.

---

[2] *The neti Pot is a small teapot that you can fill with boiling water*

and a saline solution. When the water cools to room temperature, over

I don't expect most people will want to follow a morning routine like this. However, creating a routine that works for your lifestyle can help you wake up with more energy each morning, and clear away the fog of sleep. Ideally, you'll wake up before the sunrise, but if that's not possible, a buffer of at least an hour before you have work or familial responsibilities is an excellent time to wake up.

When you wake up, instead of checking your phone or thinking about what you need to do, choose a relaxing activity like meditation or reading a book. From there, you can select some of the suggestions in this chapter to build a morning routine that works for you.

An example of a morning routine might be:
6:30: Wake up
6:30-6:45: Breathing meditation
6:45-7:15: Tea, a piece of fruit, reading a book
7:15-7:30: Self-massage

---

the sink, pour the liquid through one nostril and out the other. Repeat on the other side. This helps keep the nasal passages clear and has been very helpful to me in reducing the amount of congestion I experience. Being able to breathe deeply through your nose can help you feel calmer and relax tense muscles, which can, in turn, reduce pain. The neti pot can help you to clear your nasal passages if they are often blocked, and can be used when you have a cold to flush the sinuses.

7:30-7:45: Ayurvedic cleansing activity like a neti pot or pranayama exercise
7:45-8:00: Shower
8:00-8:15/30: yoga
8:30: Breakfast

It will take experimentation to find your ideal wake up time and morning routine. Write down what your ideal morning looks like, and adjust as you try out your routine.

Massage

Working with an experienced massage therapist can help alleviate muscle pain and tension. From an Ayurvedic perspective, you can get an Indian head massage (which involves dripping oils on your forehead), or an Ayurvedic massage, which consists in rubbing warm oils over the body. These massages can be very relaxing and help to balance the doshas.

Getting a Swedish, or deep tissue massage can get deeper into the muscle tissue to relieve pain. Working with a massage therapist who understands your condition is more important than the style of massage you choose.

Most of us can't afford to get a professional massage on a daily or weekly basis. So starting a self-massage routine in the morning can be a helpful way to start the day. I enjoy going for a massage every month or two, but in between, I try to give myself a daily massage of 10-20 minutes each morning, depending on how much time I have.

An Ayurvedic morning massage traditionally focuses on the head and neck, but I like to give myself a full body massage, or, if I'm shorter on time, focus on the areas of the body that carry the most pain and tension. I usually do the massage right before I shower so if you use any oils, you're able to clean the skin after.

The first step to starting your massage is choosing the massage oil. If you have dry skin, use heavy oil such as sesame, almond, or avocado. For sensitive skin or skin that's often red, use a cooling or neutral oil such as olive, coconut, or castor oil. For oily skin, use a light oil such as flaxseed.

Once you have your oil ready, you can heat it over the stove, or use it at room temperature. Begin with your legs, and work your way up your body all the way to your head. There are many different techniques to use for massage. I usually start with a warming rub of the area, then search out areas of tension to apply pressure to. Press into the tight spots for 5-10 seconds, and then massage around the muscle. It's hard to injure yourself or do harm with a self-massage, so really anything that feels good to you can help relieve stress and pain.

If you do see a massage therapist semi-regularly, you can ask for help creating a daily self-massage routine for in-between professional massages.

Food

Food can have a significant impact on your health: both positive and negative. I was hesitant to include it in this book because it is such a vast subject, and because it can be emotionally charged for many people.

There are so many different diets (and I specifically called this section food because I hate the word diet) that figuring out what to eat can be overwhelming. Not to mention the shame-based way we think about diet and weight in modern society.

I do think food can be a massive tool for improving your health. I do not think anyone should feel bad about their weight, severely restrict their eating, or try a new crash or fad diet to try to lose weight. One great thing that's come out of my healing journey is that I appreciate my body for what it can do, not for how it looks.

That being said, here are a few of my recommendations on what to eat:

Ayurvedic Food Recommendations

Vata is related to the element of air. When vata is in excess, this can lead to symptoms such as bloating, gassiness, diarrhoea, and constipation. To combat these effects, Ayurveda recommends consuming warm and nourishing foods and staying away from raw foods like smoothies and salads. Stick to warm soups, curries, rice dishes, and cooked vegetables.

Healthy fats and oils are recommended for decreasing vata dosha, and even a sweetener such as honey can be used in a hot ginger tea. Rice and wheat are considered the best grains for vata imbalance, while the best fruits are those that are denser, such as bananas, avocados, mangoes, berries, and figs. Minimize bean consumption, as beans can cause gas. But cheese lovers can rejoice because dairy is recommended for balancing vata!

General Diet Recommendations

Many people living with Fibromyalgia have food intolerances or sensitivities. Finding out what these are and eliminating them (or radically reducing them) in your diet, can help you feel better. For several years, I eliminated gluten and dairy and restricted eggs. Now that I'm in recovery, I'm able to eat those products occasionally but can feel the negative effects they have on my body when I eat them.

To find out if you have food intolerances, it's best to work with a dietician. They can give you a blood test to check for certain allergies and conditions like celiac disease. You can also try an elimination diet with a dietician or on your own if you're not able to work with a professional. In an elimination diet, you remove anything from your diet that could be causing you symptoms. The most common things to eliminate are: Dairy, wheat, rye, spelt, gluten, eggs, citrus fruits, caffeine, alcohol, sugar, soy, peanuts, corn, packaged/processed foods, nightshade vegetables, and anything else you suspect may be causing you digestive issues.

You should cut *all* these foods out for three weeks. It can take the body that amount of time just to eliminate the food currently in the digestive tract. Some people feel so good after these three weeks, they don't even move to the re-introduction stage!

To finish the elimination diet, try eating one of the eliminated foods on each day, over the next three to four weeks. Do not try more than one food in one day. Even if you do not have a negative reaction to a food, do not re-incorporate it into your diet until the end of the re-introduction phase. For breakfast, you should have one serving of the eliminated food, for lunch two, and dinner three. Keep a diary of how you feel after eating the food as well as how you feel the next morning. After trying each food, you can look over your notes and see if any of the foods causing you pain or digestive issues. From there, decide if you'd like to cut any foods from your diet.

If you're unsure of how to improve your diet, the best advice I've found is, "Eat food, mostly greens, not too much" by Michael Pollan. Avoid overly processed or packaged foods, cut down on processed fats and sugars, and eat at least five servings of fruits and vegetables per day.

Baths, Saunas, and Spas

Since the ancient Greeks, humans have been using water treatments to improve health. Before around 400 BC, bathing was mostly for cleansing purposes. However, the doctor Hippocrates (from the Hippocratic oath) believed that many diseases centred on an imbalance of bodily fluids.

The Greeks weren't the only ones with this idea. You may be familiar with the Japanese Ryokan, Turkish

Hammam's, or Finnish Sauna's – all water or steam-based spa treatments originating in different parts of the world.

In 2009, there was a study that found bathing in hot water could be beneficial for relieving Fibromyalgia pain. [9]

Other benefits of bathing in hot water may include:

- Helping with sleep
- Deep relaxation
- Relaxing muscles
- A supportive place to do physical activity (moving in the water is easy on the joints)

Also, the relaxing nature of spas can help activate your parasympathetic nervous system, creating a space of healing for you.

More than just the physical benefits, a nice thing about going to the spa is that it's an activity you can do with friends and family that's both fun and good for your health. Going out to bars, restaurants, or on long walks may not be possible for you with your current health challenges. But going to enjoy some hot pools and saunas is a fun activity you can do with your loved ones. My best friend and I go to a water spa a couple times a year, and after only 20 minutes of bathing in the different baths and spending quality time with my friend, I feel completely rejuvenated!

Sleep

Sleep is one of the most important tools our body has for healing. Yet, many people with chronic pain conditions struggle to sleep. People with fibromyalgia may have trouble falling asleep at night, staying asleep, and often wake up feeling unrested.

According to sleep specialists, most insomnia is caused by hyper-arousal. If you ever lie in bed feeling like your mind is racing and you can't stop thinking, this is hyper-arousal. Even if you're exhausted or feel tired all day, your mind can still be in overdrive at bedtime.

Now that we understand the role the autonomic nervous system plays in chronic pain, it's no surprise that people living with fibromyalgia also struggle to sleep. If you're in *fight or flight* mode, this is not conducive to getting a good night's sleep.

Because the reasons for poor sleep are likely linked to some of your other symptoms, everything we've covered in this book will also help you sleep better. All the systems of the body are connected, and anything we can do to help our system relax, will help both reduce pain and improve sleep.

Sleep is essential, but you also shouldn't put too much pressure on yourself to get to sleep. Often, people can feel anxious about not getting enough sleep because they know they will feel worse the next day. This anxiety makes it even harder to sleep. Then you feel even worse the next day, and it creates a vicious cycle.

Just as it's important to create a morning routine, it can also help to create an evening routine. I also like to have a plan for what to do if I can't sleep. This plan often includes doing one of the poses from my evening yoga practice in bed or doing a yoga nidra or body scan meditation.

Depending on how alert I feel, or if I get an onslaught of ideas, I might get up for an hour and do some writing or reading. This is not the best option as you will wake yourself up. But, if now and then you feel like you'd benefit by writing down all the ideas in your head, finishing something you're behind on, or picking up a book, then I say go for it. If this becomes a regular habit, you might want to re-think it. For example, if you struggle to sleep most nights, and most nights you lie in bed with your legs up the wall until you feel tired, that's a great can't-get-to-sleep plan. If once every month or two you decide to get up to finish some work or write down ideas, that is no problem. If you're getting up several nights a week to work, you won't be addressing the root of the problem and will notice a limited improvement in your sleep.

Yoga and meditation can have some of the same benefits on the brain and body as sleep can have. So if you can't sleep, doing a yoga or meditation practice is a great alternative. There's also always tomorrow night – so don't beat yourself up if you're having trouble sleeping.

There is so much to cover on the topic of sleep that I could write a whole other book on it. For now, I'll give you an overview of the top tips from a yogic perspective, and from a western scientific perspective on getting a good night's sleep:

Yogic ideas:

- Grab your massage oil and give yourself a scalp massage before bedtime.
- Eat a warm meal for dinner and avoid raw or cold foods in the evening or close to bedtime.
- Set an evening routine, and try to go to sleep around the same time every night.
- Try a restorative or yoga nidra practice in the evening or just before bed.
- Go to bed before 10:00pm and wake up before sunrise.
- Drink chamomile or valerian root tea before bed.

Western ideas:
- Turn off screens (phone, TV, laptop) two hours before bedtime. If you must look at your phone, put on a night filter to activate two hours before bedtime.
- Drink chamomile or valerian root tea before bed.
- Take a warm bath or shower before bed.
- Avoid any stimulating books, films, work, or conversations in the evening and before bed.
- Avoid caffeine at least six hours before bedtime.
- Sleep in a dark, cool room.

You don't need to do all these things but can experiment to see what works best for you and create your evening routine. An example of an evening routine could be:

6:00pm: Warm meal
7:30pm: Devices off, work for the day finished.
7:30-8:00pm: Restorative yoga or meditation practice.
8:00-8:30pm: Take a warm shower or bath.

8:30-9:00pm: Give yourself a relaxing head and scalp massage with warm oils

9:00-9:30pm: Prepare and enjoy an herbal tea. Drink the tea slowly and mindfully and perhaps enjoy reading poetry, or a book (avoiding anything stimulating such as an action-packed book or murder mystery).

9:30pm: Prepare your room for bed, closing all the curtains and lights.

9:45pm: Go to sleep.

Experiment to find a bedtime routine that works for you. If going to sleep before 10 pm sounds too early for you, try it out for one to two months. It can be difficult if you would like to spend time with friends and family in the evening. But, once you have better sleeping habits, it's easier to make exceptions to your routine. For example, I was very strict with my sleep for the first year of my recovery. Then, I started to make exceptions. If I wanted to go out with friends, I might have an afternoon nap, and then go out and enjoy. Instead of feeling guilty, I would re-commit to my healthy sleep routine the next night.

You shouldn't have to give up the things that bring you joy – joyfulness is good for your health. But if sleep is something you struggle with, it's worth it to make sleep a priority for a few months to help your body heal. Then, by paying attention to your body, you can adapt your routine to fit in other things that bring you joy.

Exercise

Yoga isn't the only form of exercise that's beneficial to chronic pain. Movement is good for your health, period.

But people living with chronic pain and fibromyalgia aren't always able to exercise. Sometimes your symptoms can get worse with exercise. One of the reasons I loved yoga when I first started practising was because it was an exercise I could do that didn't make me feel worse.

If you're at a stage where you'd like to add in other forms of exercise, then here are some tips to add it safely to your routine:

Other mindfulness-based exercises like Tai chi or Chi gong can be great places to explore if you enjoy yoga but want to try something different.

My go-to exercise is always walking. It's good for the entire body and is a low impact exercise meaning it's easy on the joints. You don't need anything to walk (other than a good pair of shoes) and can go as slow as you need to. You can start out walking 5-10 minutes a day, and gradually increase your distance each week.

As you start to feel better, you can add more intense forms of exercise. I like swimming because I used to be a swimmer, and also because swimming is another low impact exercise that's easy on the joints.

I encourage you to experiment with any exercise you like whether it's soccer, dance, running, etc. Start slow, and do each exercise mindfully, listening if your body tells you to stop.

Creativity

While everything mentioned in this chapter will help to soothe the vata dosha, you should also know that vata thrives on creativity. Help soothe the running thoughts in your mind by channelling them into a creative pursuit of journaling, painting, or photography. Taking the time to nourish your passions and artistic inspirations may help bring you into balance. Schedule time to pursue your passion.

Many people with chronic pain find that they're not able to do the things they used to do, or they can no longer pursue their passions. If you can make time to do something you're passionate about, even for just one hour a week, it can make a massive difference to your health. I know it can feel difficult to choose to do something "selfish" when you have such limited energy. You may feel like you should be doing something "practical" like cleaning the house or spending time with family members if you have the energy. But it's important to remember that we will help everyone around us, by taking care of ourselves and our health.

Action Steps

1) Create a morning and an evening routine, and commit to sticking to them for two months.
2) Pick the self-care habits (along with the yoga and meditation practices) you are most interested in trying and schedule them into your day.

Step Seven: Living Mindfully

I am currently the tallest of all my friends. I've also been this height since I was 12. When I look back through my school photos, I tower over all the other students with my poufy hair and 18-inch height difference.

I don't remember when I started hunching my shoulders. Perhaps I just had swimmers shoulders – always moving forwards in the pool. Maybe I felt self-conscious about my height and began slouching. Either way, I've had pretty terrible posture since I was a teenager. This lousy posture causes me a lot of pain in my neck and shoulders.

Once I started practising yoga and meditation, my posture began improving. I could feel relief in my neck in shoulders when I sat up straight in a meditation session. The problem was, this didn't often translate to the rest of my day. When I started developing neck and shoulder tension again recently, I realized that despite doing 5-10 hours of yoga per week, it wasn't making up for the other 30-40 hours I was spending hunched in front of a laptop, sitting in bed or on a couch to work.

I began to realize it wasn't just the physical yoga practice that I need to help my posture – it's the little decisions I make each day that will make the biggest difference. Am I going to sit at the table, or sit on the couch, placing my laptop on the coffee table? If I sit at the table am I going to sit up straight, or lean back in the chair and let my shoulders round? Am I going to commit to sitting straight, or am I going to let stress get the better of me and tell myself I'll work on my posture later, right now I need to get this work done?

When I make too many poor posture decisions during the day, it doesn't matter how often I do yoga, I'll start slouching again, and my neck and shoulder pain will come back. We've already established that a shorter, consistent yoga practice can have more power than one longer practice. It's also the small, micro health decisions we make each day that have a more significant impact on our long-term health than any major overhaul.

Living a yogic and mindful lifestyle isn't only about practising yoga and meditation – it's everything in between.

I can't count the number of times (especially when living in a bigger city), that I went to a yoga class at a studio, felt very relaxed after, and in the 45 minutes it took me to get home felt stressed again because the commute was busy. It wasn't until I started to bring my intentions from yoga class – to breathe deeply, to show compassion to others, to be present – that my stress didn't shoot back after my commute home.

Living a mindful life doesn't mean you need to walk around being zen, calm, and compassionate all the time. Just as meditating doesn't mean we need to stop thinking, being mindful doesn't mean we don't experience all the stresses of daily life, it just means we're able to come back to an oasis of calm.

For example, setting a timer on your phone to do nothing for 15-seconds, or do a short breathing meditation for two to three minutes, can make a big difference in your stress levels, and how you feel throughout the rest of the day.

Yoga and meditation aren't the only mindful activities we can do. Anything can be mindful from washing the dishes to taking a shower or talking to a friend. We need to choose to be present again and again and again.

We can eat mindfully, savouring each flavour. We can travel mindfully, enjoying each moment, experiencing a true beginner's mind every new place we go. We can be mindful in our relationships. How often do you talk with friends and family, and you've each got a smartphone on the table? We can put the phones away, the other thoughts of what we're doing later away, and be fully present in our conversations with loved ones.

All these things are micro-decisions you can make each day, but can have a significant impact on your pain and energy levels.

When we live in the moment, we are ruled less by our automatic reaction to something, and more by the choices we make. We can choose to be compassionate and kind to ourselves as much as we are to our loved ones and to those who might bother or annoy us as much as we are to ourselves.

We can choose to have gratitude for the things we have, even when it feels like there is so much we don't have to be grateful for. When you're living mindfully, you can choose to be grateful for the taste of food, or the time you got to spend with a friend. You can choose to be fully present during each interaction or life experience. In other words, you can fully show up for your life.

We can also choose to find joy in our lives. To do the things we love. To explore creativity. To watch the ebb and flow of our pain, and know it is not permanent. Despite our pain, we can find the joy in each moment, as it is.

Thank You!

I hope you've enjoyed this book and you now have some concrete ideas on how yoga can help you recover from chronic pain. If you enjoyed this book, I would love it if you could leave a review on amazon.com or goodreads.com. Your honest review will help me get this information out to more people living with chronic pain! If you have any questions about anything in this book, or would like to update me on your progress, I'd love to hear from you at kayla@arogayoga.com!

For more information on yoga for chronic illness, sign up for my newsletter at www.arogayoga.com where I post bi-monthly blog posts and free videos.

About the Author

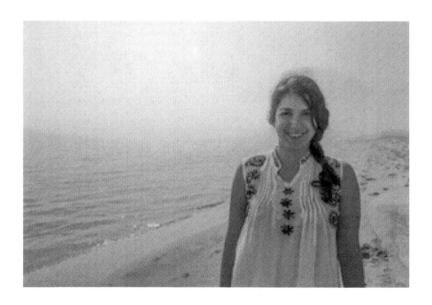

Kayla Kurin is the author of 'Yoga for Chronic Pain: 7 steps to aid recovery from Fibromyalgia'. Kayla is a yoga therapist, writer, and constant traveller who is always ready to embark on her next adventure and share what she's learned with humour, compassion, and kindness. You can learn more about her on her website: arogayoga.com.

Yoga for Chronic Fatigue Preview

"You may not control all the events that happen to you, but you can decide not to be reduced by them."- Maya Angelou, Letters To My Daughter.

I don't remember everything about the year I started to develop Chronic Fatigue Syndrome. I was so young that it came in a blur. I can only distinguish between the 'before time' because I remember how into sports I was. I swam competitively and was on every school sports team (my favourites were volleyball, basketball, and softball). I had swimming practice almost every day, and for the few years I had been on the team I was steadily improving. Until I wasn't.

I had been excited to go to practices before but now getting in the water after a day of school felt exhausting. My body felt heavy like it couldn't glide through the water anymore. My limbs didn't want to do much more than float. I had never been a morning person but now getting up for school was impossible. I might have stayed up until 4am the night before if I had slept at all (and I often woke up feeling like I hadn't). I would 'clue out' for long periods of the day, not sure what the teacher had said. Or I'd read the same paragraph of text over and over again without taking in any of the information. It was clear that something was wrong, I just didn't know what.

We've all had days where we wake up feeling tired. But if you're living with Chronic Fatigue Syndrome (CFS), you might have forgotten what it's like to wake up without feeling tired. "Normal" fatigue might be relieved by rest, sleep, caffeine, or removing an underlying cause such as a viral illness. Yet, the exhaustion that comes with Chronic Fatigue Syndrome sticks around no matter what treatments sufferers try.

To complicate matters, despite the name, CFS is more than just fatigue. It's persistent fatigue that lasts more than 6 months, is accompanied by decreased mental functioning[10], and often includes symptoms such as joint pain, trouble sleeping (insomnia), sore throat, lowered or heightened immune function, and sometimes depression as a result of the loss of quality of life.

Chronic Fatigue Syndrome has had a controversial history in the medical community. For many years, patients weren't believed about the severity of their symptoms. Even now, many patients are misdiagnosed with depression[11], or, told it's "all in their head". I was fortunate that over 15 years ago, I got a diagnosis within 6 months. However, after getting that diagnosis, my doctor didn't know what to do with me. I got passed around to different specialists, and yes, often got treated for depression. I was told to drink caffeine if I felt tired or try to push through, and went on a carousel of sleeping pills that never seemed to work for any lasting period of time.

Yet, in the past decade research around CFS has improved, and the scientific community has a better idea of what the illness is. CFS is now classified as a neurological disorder involving the central nervous system (CNS) and peripheral nervous system (PNS). The PNS includes the autonomic nervous system which we'll explore in depth in this book.

While no one knows for sure what causes chronic fatigue syndrome, we do have a better understanding of what this illness looks like in the body. This may help you better understand your fatigue, and also understand how practices like yoga can help you decrease your fatigue. While there are no consistent biomarkers for diagnosing CFS, Anthony L. Komaroff argues in his 2017 study that there are signs that an imbalanced CNS can cause chronic fatigue syndrome. Many studies have found an increase in stress hormones in patients with CFS, as well as reduced levels of antioxidants, and the lack of ability to recover from minor illnesses. [12]

What we don't know the answer to is the question of: which came first? Do these physiological symptoms cause the illness? Or does the illness produce the physiological symptoms? However, even though we don't know the answer to that question, getting a better understanding of what is going on in the bodies of people living with CFS is helpful to understanding how we can ease our bodies into recovery mode.

Western treatment for CFS is lacking. Since there is no known cause and it's not a life-threatening illness, this illness has not been a priority in the medical community. There are no medications doctors can prescribe to patients with CFS. Depending on your doctor, you may get told something along the lines of, "it's all in your head, see a shrink" or find a doctor who tries to treat specific symptoms like poor sleep without addressing the underlying causes of the illness. If you're lucky, you'll have found a doctor who is willing to take a holistic approach to recovery from CFS.

I do believe that there are many tools we can use from western medicine to aid our healing, and temporary fixes like sleeping pills can be very helpful for people with severe symptoms for the short term. But, in the long run, if we don't fully heal our bodies, we'll have to continue treating the symptoms forever. Some doctors are now beginning to recommend complementary treatments such as yoga, meditation, or massage. But, many patients are left on their own.

While there are some significant gaps in western medicine, specifically when it comes to dealing with a chronic illness like CFS, we shouldn't discount the rigorous research practices applied to western medical practices. We should use these resources when it makes sense to our healthcare team and us. Universal healing strategies like deep breathing, exercise, and diet can be used in conjunction with specific healing strategies like medication or surgery.

I will always refer to my yoga practice as holistic or complementary. It adds to the care I receive from my doctors but does not replace it. I've been able to help many people feel better, sleep better, and have more energy in my yoga practice, but I am not a doctor and don't give medical advice. The most successful cases I've seen are the ones where my student is also working with a physician who understands the power of complementary medicine and meditation.

High Sensitivity

One consideration when thinking about CFS is high sensitivity. The book *The Highly Sensitive Person* by Elaine Aron dives into this topic in depth, and I recommend reading this book if you identify as a sensitive person! I didn't think of myself as a sensitive person before reading this book (I was tough enough to defeat a death eater, indeed), but this book changed my understanding of what sensitivity means. While it does refer to emotional sensitivity, and it does seem like people with CFS do have stronger emotional reactions[13] than the average population, sensitivity refers to a host of things that are out of our control.

Sensitivity may refer to sensitivity to light and sound, sensitivity to people (being introverted), sensitivity to air quality, sensitivity to food, and any other emotional or environmental factors.

If you find that you get drained by city life or being around people quicker than your friends and family, you may be a highly sensitive person (HSP).

This high sensitivity could mean that you're more affected by environmental factors than your peers, which will set off that sympathetic nervous system and leave you feeling drained. Repeating this cycle over many years may mirror many of the symptoms of chronic fatigue syndrome.

While we don't know for sure what causes CFS, we do know some of the related physiological factors that make it harder for us to heal. By using various techniques to soothe the nervous system and build a life that factors in our sensitivity, we can begin on the path to recovery.

Being sick with a chronic illness requires you to become a detective. You need to search for clues to what is making your symptoms worse and be on high alert for the things that make you feel better. By drawing awareness to the things we do know, we can start creating a blueprint to feeling better.

Read Yoga for Chronic Fatigue: 7 Steps to Aid Recovery From Chronic Fatigue Syndrome with Yoga on Amazon, Kobo, or Apple Books!

Endnotes

[1] Aaron A. Hanyu-Deutmeyer;Scott C. Dulebohn *Pain, Phantom Limb* (Statpearls: April 17, 2018:
https://www.ncbi.nlm.nih.gov/books/NBK448188/)
[2] . Sympathetic Nervous System Indeed!... And Why Some People Suffer Over Your Pain (Bodyinmind.org August 2017:
https://bodyinmind.org/meaning-pain-giummarra/)
3. Lara Hilton et al. *Mindfulness Meditation for Chronic Pain: Systemic Review and Meta-analysis* (Annals of Behavioral Medicine 2017; 51(2): 199–213:
https://www.ncbi.nlm.nih.gov/pmc/articles/PMC5368208/)
4. Chris C. Streeter at al. *Effects of Yoga Versus Walking on Mood, Anxiety, and Brain GABA levels* (Journal of Alternative and Complementary Medicine 2010 Nov; 16(11): 1145–1152:
https://www.ncbi.nlm.nih.gov/pmc/articles/PMC3111147/)

[5] Turan, B., Foltz, C., Cavanagh, J. F., Wallace, B. A., Cullen, M., Rosenberg, E. L., Jennings, P., Ekman, P., & Kemeny, M. E. (2015).Anticipatory Sensitization to Repeated Stressors: the role of initital cortisol reactivity and meditation/emotion skills training.Psychoneuroendocrinology, 52, 229-238

6. Ankad RD et al. *Effect of short-term Pranayama and Meditation on Cardiovascular Functions in Healthy Individuals* (Heart Views 2011 Apr;12(2):58-62:
https://www.ncbi.nlm.nih.gov/pubmed/22121462)

Matarelli D, Cocchioni M, Scuri S, Pompei P. *Diaphragmatic Breathing Reduce Postprandial Oxidative Stress* (J Altern Complement Med. 2011 Jul;17(7):623-8:
https://www.ncbi.nlm.nih.gov/pubmed/21688985

[7] Alyson Ross et al. Evid Based Complement Alternat Med. 2012; 2012: 983258.
Published online 2012 Aug 14.doi:10.1155/2012/983258

[8] Ranganathan VK1,Siemionow V,Liu JZ,Sahgal V,Yue GH
Neuropsychologia.2004;42(7):944-56.

9. Francon A, Forestier R. *Spa Therapy in Rheumatology* (Bull Acad Natl Med.2009 Jun;193(6):1345-56: https://www.ncbi.nlm.nih.gov/pubmed/20120164)

[10] Jefferson R Roberts, Chronic Fatigue Syndrome (CFS), https://emedicine.medscape.com/article/235980-overview.

[11] James P Griffith, Fahd A Zarrouf, A Systemic Review of Chronic Fatigue Syndrome: Don't Assume It's Depression, Prim Care Companion J Clin Psychiatry. 2008; 10(2): 120–128.

[12] Anthony L. Komaroff. Inflammation correlates with symptoms in chronic fatigue syndrome. PNASAugust 22, 2017114(34)8914-8916;published ahead of print August 15, 2017https://doi.org/10.1073/pnas.1712475114

[13] Rimes, K. A., Ashcroft, J., Bryan, L., & Chalder, T. (2016). Emotional suppression in chronic fatigue syndrome: Experimental study.Health Psychology, 35(9), 979-986. http://dx.doi.org/10.1037/hea0000341

Made in the USA
San Bernardino, CA
07 December 2019